The Definitive Plant-Based Dinner Recipe Book

An Amazing Collection of Healthy Recipes to Discover the Benefits of a Plant-Based Diet

I0222580

Dave Ingram

Table of contents

Mom's Famous Chili

Preparation Time: 10 minutes

Cooking Time: 10 minutes

Servings: 4

Ingredients:

1 pound red black beans, soaked overnight and drained

3 tablespoons olive oil

1 large red onion, diced 2 bell peppers, diced

1 poblano pepper, minced

1   large carrot, trimmed and diced 2 cloves garlic, minced

2   bay leaves

1   teaspoon mixed peppercorns

Kosher salt and cayenne pepper, to taste 1 tablespoon paprika

2   ripe tomatoes, pureed

2 tablespoons tomato ketchup 3 cups vegetable broth

Directions:

1.   Cover the soaked beans with a fresh change of cold water and bring to a boil. Let it boil for about 10 minutes. Turn the heat to a simmer and continue to cook for 50 to 55 minutes or until tender.

2.   Sauté the onion, peppers, and carrot to hot oil.

3.   Sauté the garlic for about 30 seconds or until aromatic.

4.   Add in the remaining ingredients along with the cooked beans. Let it simmer, stirring periodically, for 25 to 30 minutes or until cooked through.

5.   Discard the bay leaves, ladle into individual bowls and serve hot!

Nutrition: Calories: 455, Fat: 10.5g, Carbs: 68.6g, Protein: 24.7g

Creamed Chickpea Salad with Pine Nuts

Preparation Time: 10 minutes

Cooking Time: 10 minutes

Servings: 4

Ingredients:

16 oz. canned chickpeas, drained 1 teaspoon garlic, minced

1 shallot, chopped

1 cup cherry tomatoes, halved 1 bell pepper, seeded and sliced 1/4 cup fresh basil, chopped 1/4 cup fresh parsley, chopped 1/2 cup vegan mayonnaise

1 tablespoon lemon juice 1 teaspoon capers, draineds

Salt and pepper, to taste 2 oz. pine nuts

Directions:

1.   Place the chickpeas, vegetables, and herbs in a salad bowl.

2.   Add in the mayonnaise, lemon juice, capers, salt, and black pepper. Stir to combine.

3.   Top with pine nuts and serve immediately.

Nutrition: Calories: 386, Fat: 22.5g, Carbs: 37.2g, Protein: 12.9g

Black Bean Buda Bowl

Preparation Time: 10 minutes

Cooking Time: 10 minutes

Servings: 4

Ingredients:

1/2 pound beans, soaked and drained 2 cups brown rice, cooked

1 medium-sized onion, thinly sliced 1 cup bell pepper, seeded and sliced 1 jalapeno pepper, seeded and sliced 2 cloves garlic, minced

1 cup arugula

1 cup baby spinach 1 teaspoon lime zest

1 tablespoon Dijon mustard 1/4 cup red wine

1/4 cup e.v.o. oil 2 tablespoons agave syrup

Flaky sea salt and ground black pepper, to taste 1/4 cup fresh Italian parsley, roughly chopped

Directions:

1.   Cover the soaked beans with a fresh change of cold water and bring to a boil. Let it boil for about 10 minutes. Turn the heat to a simmer and continue to cook for 50 to 55 minutes or until tender.

2.   To serve, divide the beans and rice between serving bowls; top with the vegetables.

3.   A small mixing dish thoroughly combines the lime zest, mustard, vinegar, olive oil, agave syrup, salt, and pepper. Drizzle the vinaigrette over the salad.

4.   Garnish with fresh Italian parsley.

Nutrition: Calories: 365, Fat: 14.1g, Carbs: 45.6g, Protein: 15.5g

Middle Eastern Chickpea Stew

Preparation Time: 10 minutes

Cooking Time: 10 minutes

Servings: 4

Ingredients

1 onion

1 chili pepper

2 garlic cloves

1 teaspoon mustard seeds 1 teaspoon coriander seeds 1 bay leaf

1/2 cup tomato puree 2 tablespoons olive oil

1   celery with leaves, chopped

2   medium carrots, trimmed and chopped 2 cups vegetable broth

1 teaspoon ground cumin

1 small-sized cinnamon stick

16 oz. canned chickpeas, drained

2 cups Swiss chard, torn into pieces

Directions:

1.   In your blender or food processor, blend the onion, chili pepper, garlic, mustard seeds, coriander seeds, bay leaf, and tomato puree into a paste.

2.   In a stockpot, heat the olive oil until sizzling. Now, cook the celery and carrots for about 3 minutes or until they've softened. Add in the paste and continue to cook for a further 2 minutes.

3.   Then, add vegetable broth, cumin, cinnamon, and chickpeas; bring it to a gentle boil.

4.   Turn the heat to simmer and let it cook for 6 minutes; fold in Swiss chard and continue to cook for 4 to 5 minutes more or until the leaves wilt. Serve hot and enjoy!

Nutrition: Calories: 305, Fat: 11.2g, Carbs: 38.6g, Protein: 12.7g

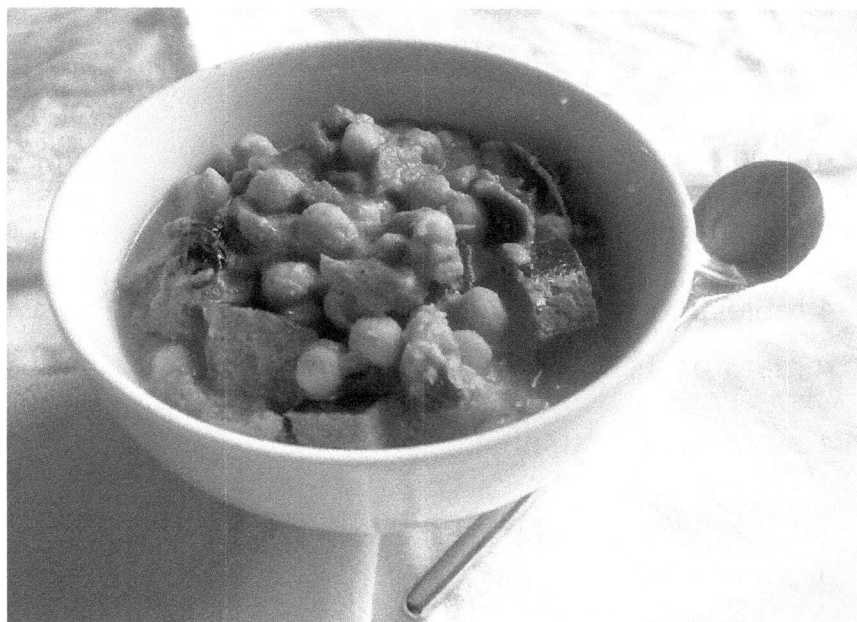

Lentil and Tomato Dip

Preparation Time: 10 minutes

Cooking Time: 10 minutes

Servings: 4

Ingredients:

16 oz. lentils, boiled and drained

4 tablespoons sun-dried tomatoes, chopped 1 cup tomato paste

4 tablespoons tahini

1   teaspoon stone-ground mustard 1 teaspoon ground cumin

1/4 teaspoon ground bay leaf 1 teaspoon red pepper flakes

Salt and pepper, to taste

Directions:

1.   Blitz all the ingredients in your blender or food processor until your desired consistency is reached.

2.   Place in your refrigerator until ready to serve.

3.   Serve with toasted pita wedges or vegetable sticks. Enjoy!

Nutrition: Calories: 144, Fat: 4.5g, Carbs: 20.2g, Protein: 8.1g

Creamed Green Pea Salad

Preparation Time: 10 minutes

Cooking Time: 10 minutes

Servings: 4

Ingredients:

2   (14.5 oz.) cans green peas, drained

 1/2 cup vegan mayonnaise 1 teaspoon Dijon mustard

2 tablespoons scallions, chopped 2 pickles, chopped

1/2 cup marinated mushrooms, chopped and drained 1/2 teaspoon garlic, minced

Salt and pepper, to taste

Directions:

1.   Place all the ingredients in a salad bowl. Gently stir to combine.

2.   Place the salad in your refrigerator until ready to serve.

Nutrition: Calories: 154, Fat: 6.7g, Carbs: 17.3g, Protein: 6.9g

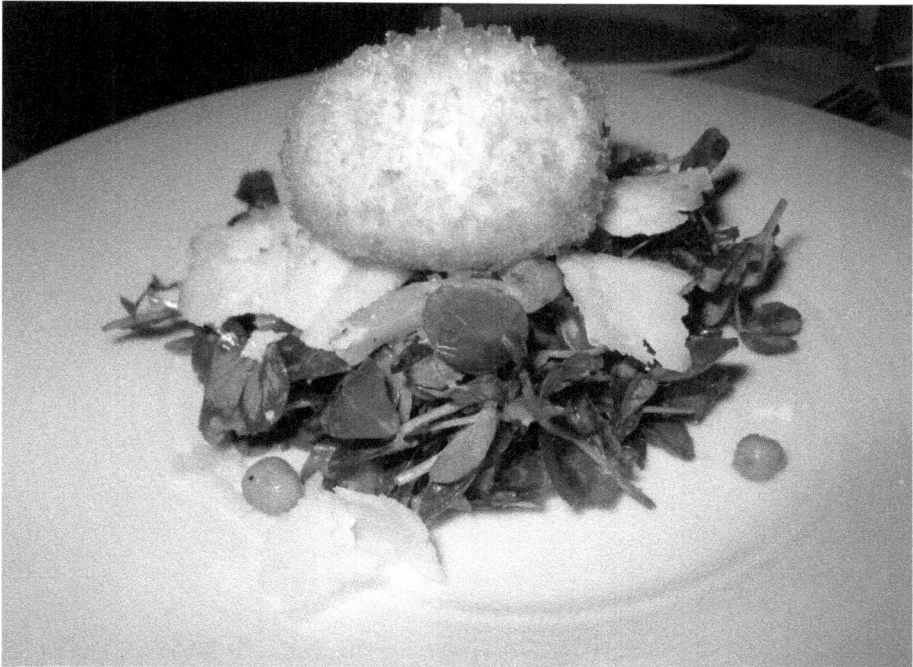

Cashew Zucchinis

Preparation Time: 10 minutes

Cooking Time: 40 minutes

Servings: 4

Ingredients:

1 pound zucchinis, sliced

½ cup cashews, soaked and drained

1   cup coconut milk

¼ teaspoon nutmeg, ground 1 teaspoon chili powder

A pinch of salt and black pepper

Directions:

1.   In a roasting pan, mix the zucchinis with the cashews and the other ingredients, toss gently, and cook at 380 degrees F for 40 minutes.

2.   Divide into bowls and serve.

Nutrition: calories 200 fat 5 fiber 3 carbs 7.1 protein 6.5

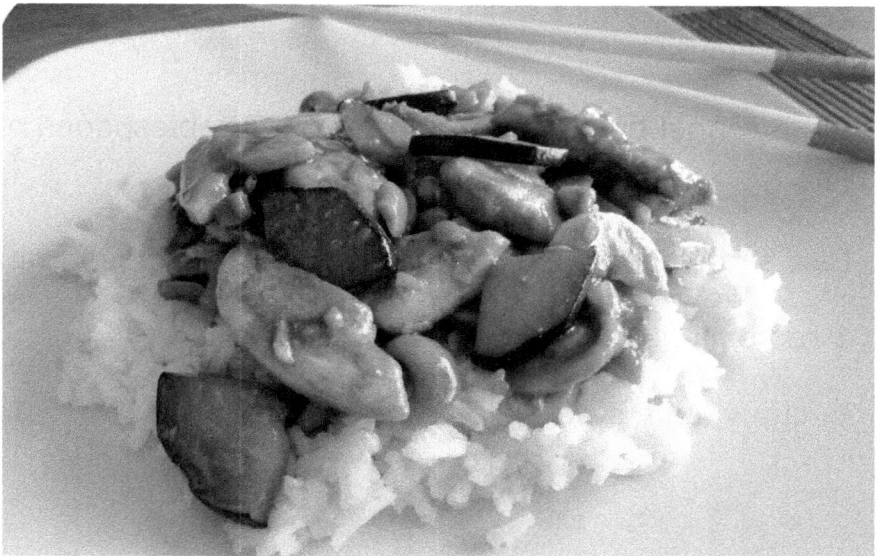

Chili Fennel

Preparation Time: 10 minutes

Cooking Time: 8 minutes

Servings: 4

Ingredients:

2   fennel bulbs, cut into quarters 3 tablespoons olive oil

Salt and black pepper to the taste 1 garlic clove, minced

1 red chili pepper, chopped

¾ cup veggie stock Juice of ½ lemon

Directions:

1.   Heat a pan that fits your Air Fryer with the oil over medium-high heat, add garlic and chili pepper, stir and cook for 2 minutes.

2.   Add fennel, salt, pepper, stock, and lemon juice, toss to coat, introduce in your Air Fryer, and cook at 350 ° F for at least 6 minutes.

3.   Divide into plates and serve as a side dish.

Nutrition: Calories: 158 kcal Protein: 3.57 g Fat: 11.94 g Carbohydrates: 11.33 g

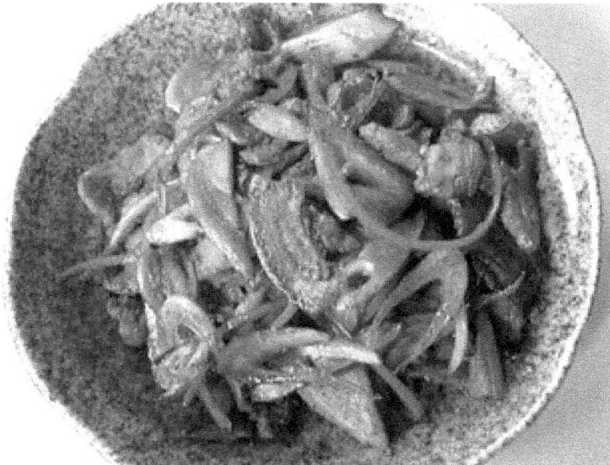

Collard Greens and Tomatoes

Preparation Time: 10 minutes

Cooking Time: 10 minutes

Servings: 9

Ingredients:

1 pound collard greens

¼ cup cherry tomatoes halved 1 tablespoon apple cider vinegar 2 tablespoons veggie stock

Salt and black pepper to the taste

Directions:

1.   Combine tomatoes, collard greens, vinegar, stock, salt, and pepper in a pan, stir, introduce in your Air Fryer and cook at 320 ° F for 10 minutes.

2.   Divide between plates and serve as a side dish.

Nutrition: Calories: 28 kcal Protein: 2.34 g Fat: 0.99 g
Carbohydrates: 3.26 g

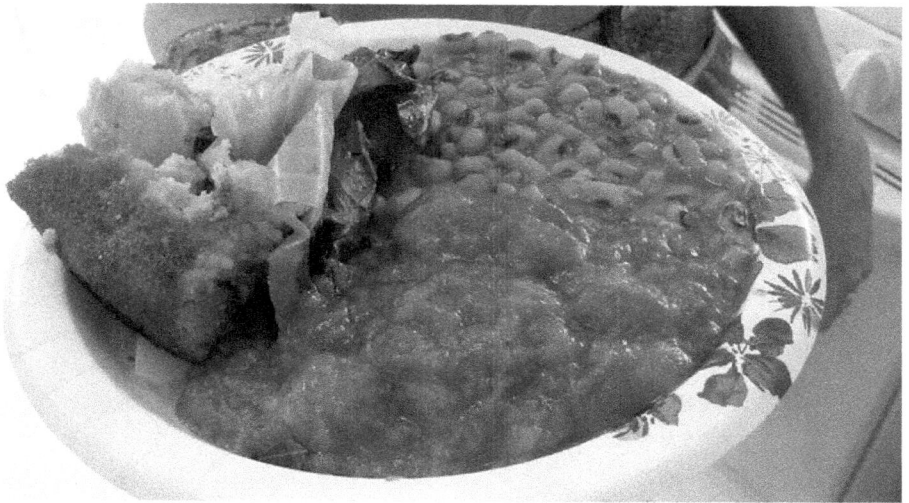

Bean and Carrot Spirals

Preparation Time: 10 minutes

Cooking Time: 40 minutes

Servings: 24

Ingredients:

4 8-inch flour tortillas

1 ½ cups of Easy Mean White Bean dip 10 ounces spinach leaves

½ cup diced carrots

½ cup diced red peppers

Directions:

1.   Starts by preparing the bean dip, seen above. Next, spread out the bean dip on each tortilla, making sure to leave about a ¾ inch white border on the tortillas' surface. Next, place spinach in the center of the tortilla, followed by carrots and red peppers.

2.   Roll the tortillas into tight rolls, and cover every roll with plastic wrap or aluminum foil.

3.   Let them chill in the fridge for twenty-four hours.

4.   Afterward, remove the wrap from the spirals and remove the very ends of the rolls. Slice the rolls into six individual spiral pieces, and arrange them on a platter for serving. Enjoy!

Nutrition: Calories: 205 kcal Protein: 6.41 g Fat: 4.16 g Carbohydrates: 35.13 g

Tofu Nuggets with Barbecue Glaze

Preparation Time: 10 minutes

Cooking Time: 25 minutes

Servings: 9

Ingredients:

32 ounces tofu

1 cup quick vegan barbecue sauce

Directions:

1.   Set the oven to 425F.

2.   Next, slice the tofu and blot the tofu with clean towels. Next, slice and dice the tofu and eliminate the water from the tofu material.

3.   Stir the tofu with the vegan barbecue sauce, and place the tofu on a baking sheet.

4.   Bake the tofu for fifteen minutes. Afterward, stir the tofu and bake the tofu for an additional ten minutes.

5.   Enjoy!

Nutrition: Calories: 311 kcal Protein: 19.94 g Fat: 21.02 g Carbohydrates: 15.55 g

Peppered Pinto Beans

Preparation Time: 10 minutes

Cooking Time: 15 minutes

Servings: 6

Ingredients:

1 tsp. Chili powder 1 tsp. ground cumin

.5 cup Vegetable 2 cans Pinto beans 1 Minced jalapeno

1 Diced red bell pepper 1 tsp. Olive oil

Directions:

1.   Take out a pot and heat the oil. Cook the jalapeno and pepper for a bit before adding in the pepper, salt, cumin, broth, and beans.

2.   Place to a boil and then reduce the heat to cook for a bit. After 10 minutes, let it cool and serve.

Nutrition: Calories: 183 Carbs: 32g Fat: 2g Protein: 11g

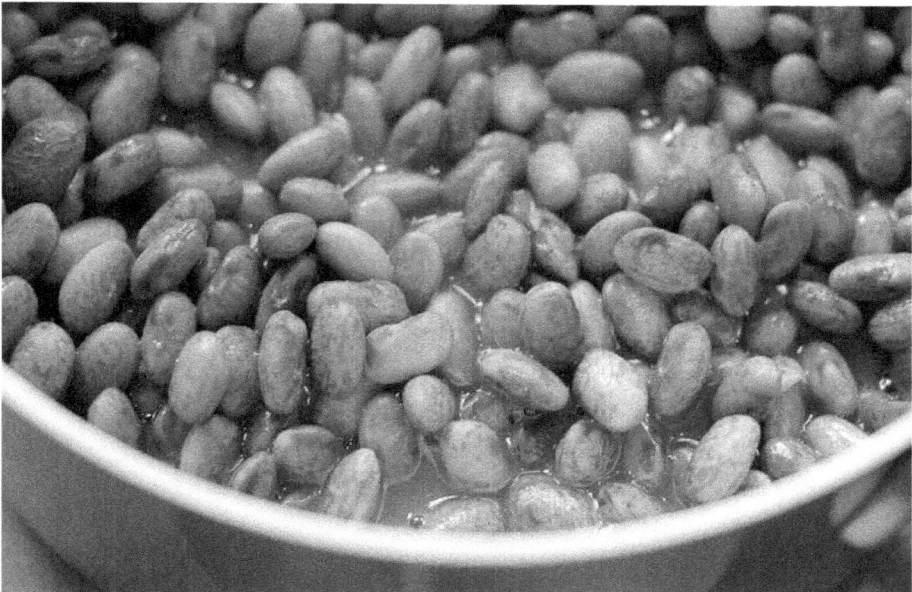

Pesto and White Bean Pasta

Preparation Time: 10 minutes

Cooking Time: 10 minutes

Servings: 4

Ingredients:

5 cup Chopped black olives

.25 Diced red onion

1 cup Chopped tomato

.5 cup Spinach pesto

1.5   cup Cannellini beans 8 oz. Rotini pasta, cooked

Directions:

1.   Bring out a bowl and toss together the pesto, beans, and pasta.

2.   Add in the olives, red onion, and tomato and toss around a bit more before serving.

Nutrition: Calories 544 Carbs 83g Fat 17g Protein 23g

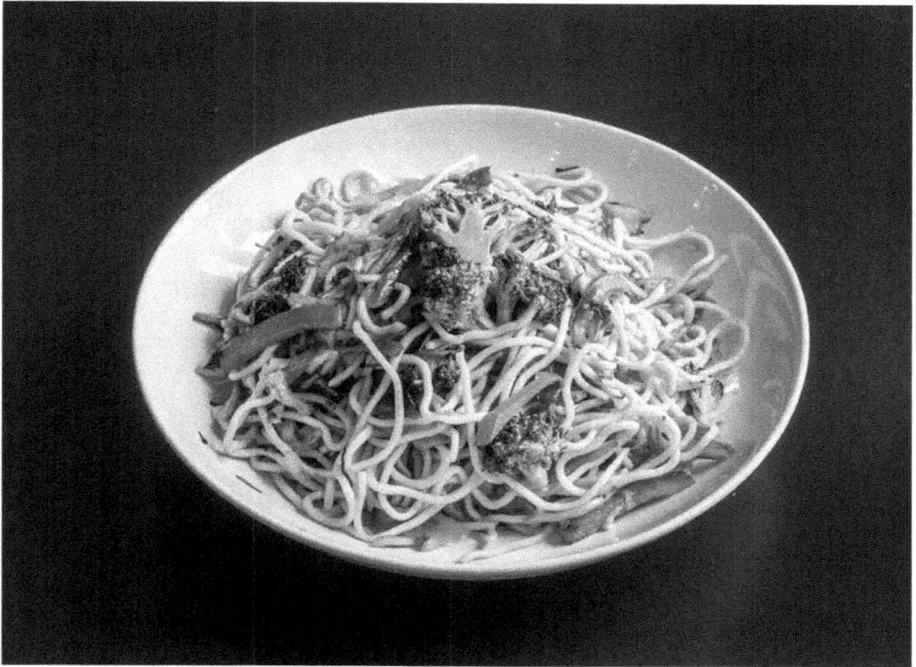

Baked Okra and Tomato

Preparation Time: 10 minutes

Cooking Time: 75 minutes

Servings: 6

Ingredients:

½ cup lima beans, frozen 4 tomatoes, chopped

8 ounces okra, fresh and washed, stemmed, sliced into ½ inch thick slices

1 onion, sliced into rings

½ sweet pepper, seeded and sliced thin Pinch of crushed red pepper

Salt to taste

Directions:

1.   Preheat your oven to 350 degrees Fahrenheit

2.   Cook lima beans in water accordingly and drain them; take a 2quart casserole tin

3.   Add all listed ingredients to the dish and cover with foil, bake for 45 minutes

4.   Uncover the dish, stir well and bake for 35 minutes more

5.   Stir, then serve, and enjoy!

Nutrition: Calories: 55 Fat: 0g Carbohydrates: 12g Protein: 3g

Curried Apple

Preparation Time: 10 minutes

Cooking Time: 90 minutes

Servings: 4

Ingredients:

1   tablespoon fresh lemon juice

½ cup of water

2   apples, Fuji or Honeycrisp, cored and thinly sliced into rings 1 teaspoon curry powder

Directions:

1.   Set the oven to 200F, take a rimmed baking sheet, and line with parchment paper

2.   Take a bowl and mix in lemon juice and water, add apples and soak for 2 minutes

3.   Pat them dry and arrange in a single layer on your baking sheet, dust curry powder on top of apple slices

4.   Bake for 45 minutes. After 45 minutes, turn the apples and bake for 45 minutes more

5.   Let them cool for extra crispiness, serve and enjoy!

Nutrition: Calories: 240 Fat: 13g Carbohydrates: 20g Protein: 6g

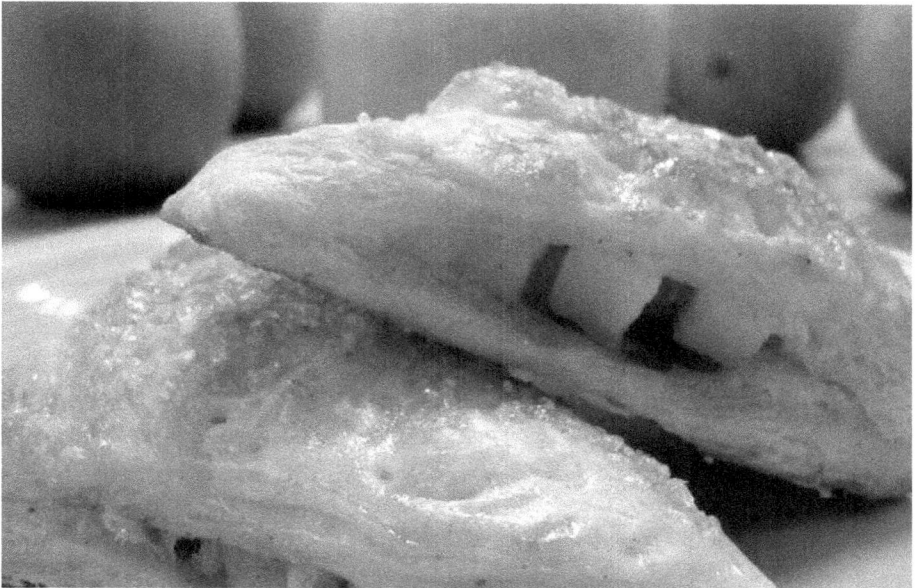

Wild Rice and Millet Croquettes

Preparation Time: 5 minutes

Cooking Time: 20 minutes

Servings: 4

Ingredients:

¾ cooked millet

½ cup cooked wild rice

3   tablespoons extra virgin olive oil

¼ cup onion, minced

1 celery rib, finely minced

¼ cup carrot, shredded 1/3 cup all-purpose flour

¼ cup fresh parsley, chopped 2 teaspoons dried dill weed Salt and pepper to taste

Directions:

1.   Add cooked millet and wild rice to a large-sized bowl, keep it to one side

2. Take a medium skillet and add 1 tablespoon of oil, place it over medium heat

3. Put onion, celery, and carrot and cook for at least 5 minutes

4. Add veggies and stir in flour, parsley, salt, pepper, and dill weed

5. Mix well and transfer to the fridge, let it sit for 20 minutes

6. Use hands to shape mixture into small patties, take a large skillet and place it over medium heat

7. Add 2 tablespoons of oil and let it heat up

8. Add croquettes and cook for 8 minutes in total until golden brown

9. Serve and enjoy!

Nutrition: Calories: 250 Fat: 9g Carbohydrates: 33g Protein: 9g

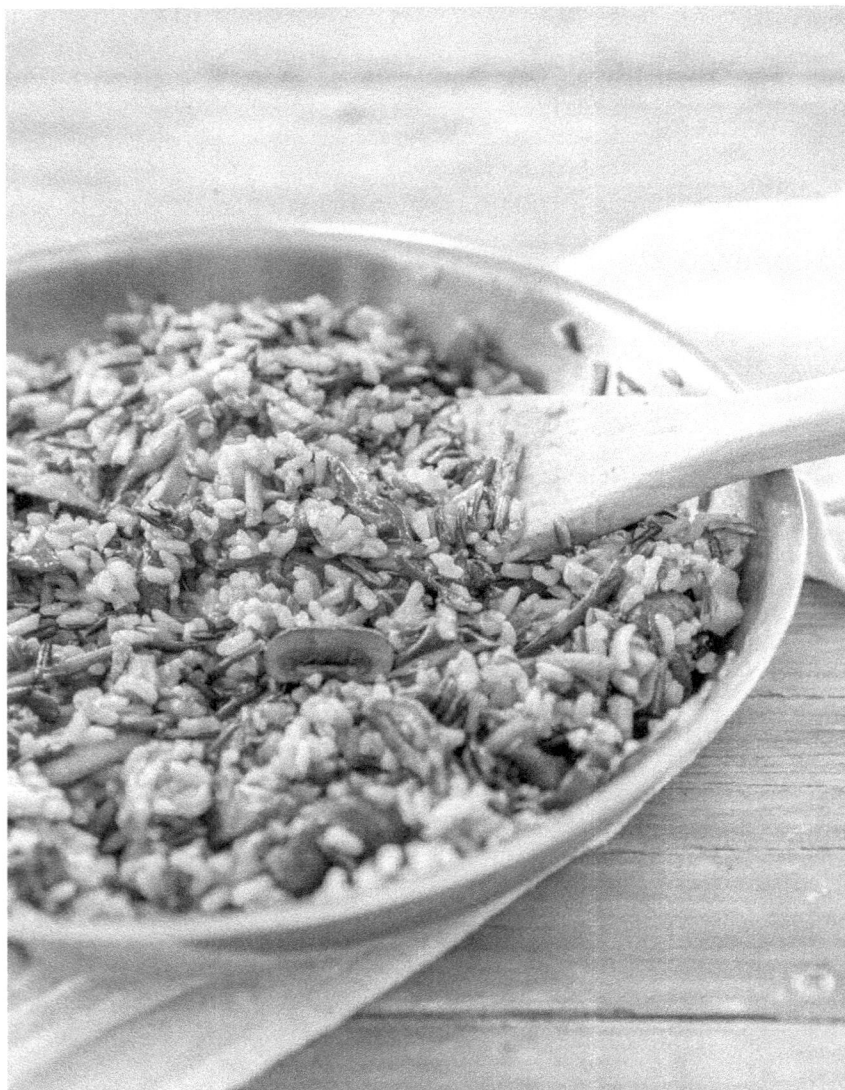

Grilled Eggplant Steaks

Preparation Time: 10 minutes

Cooking Time: 10 minutes

Servings: 4

Ingredients:

4 Roma tomatoes, diced 8 ounces cashew cream 2 eggplants

1 tablespoon olive oil 1 cup parsley, chopped 1 cucumber, diced

Salt and pepper to taste

Directions:

1.   Slice eggplants into three thick steaks, drizzle with oil, and season with salt and pepper

2.   Grill in a pan for 4 minutes per side

3.   Top with remaining ingredients

4.   Serve and enjoy!

Nutrition: Calories: 86 Fat: 7g Carbohydrates: 12g
Protein: 8g

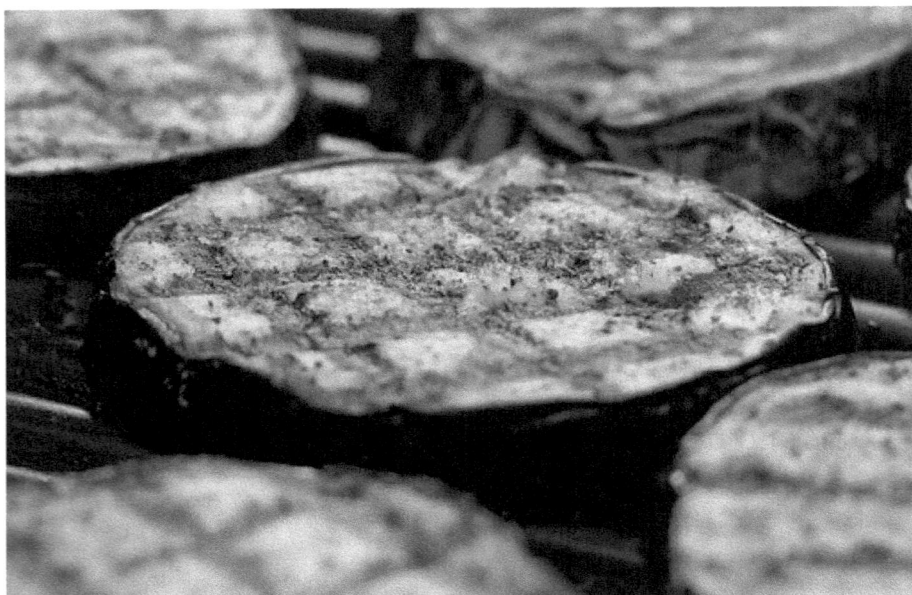

Glazed Avocado

Preparation Time: 10 minutes

Cooking Time: 12 minutes

Servings: 4

Ingredients:

1 tablespoon stevia 1 teaspoon olive oil 1 teaspoon water

1   teaspoon lemon juice

½ teaspoon rosemary, dried

½ teaspoon ground black pepper

2   avocados, peeled, pitted, and cut into large pieces

Directions:

1.   Heat a pan with the oil over medium heat, add the avocados, stevia, and the other ingredients, toss, cook for 12 minutes, divide into bowls and serve.

Nutrition: calories 262 fat 9.6 fiber 0.1 carbs 6.5 protein 7.9

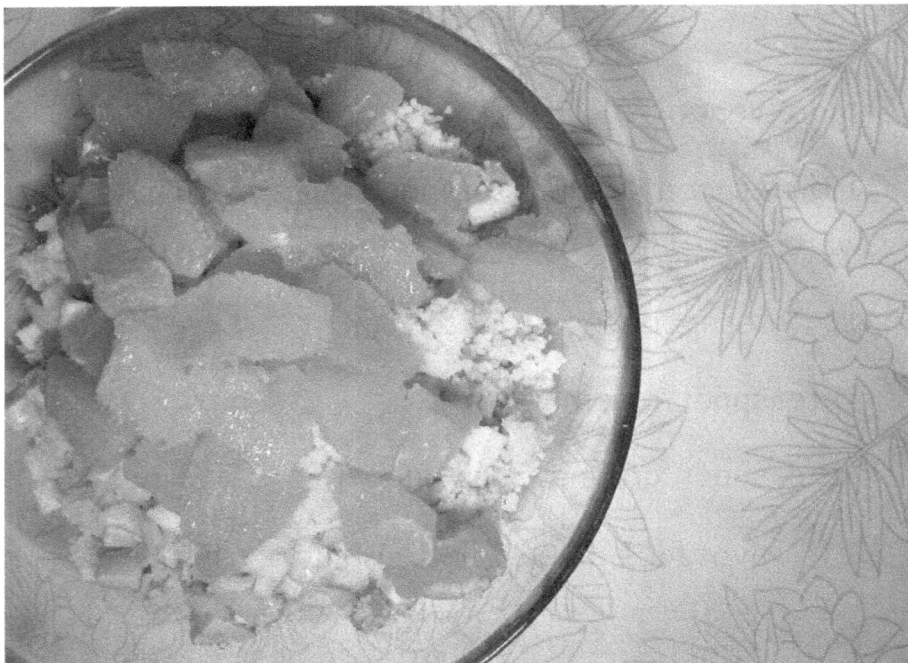

Green Lentil Stew with Collard Greens

Preparation Time: 10 minutes

Cooking Time: 10 minutes

Servings: 4

Ingredients:

2   tablespoons olive oil 1 onion, chopped

2 potatoes

1 bell pepper, chopped

2 carrots, chopped

1 parsnip, chopped

1   celery, chopped

2   cloves garlic

1 ½ cups green lentils

1 tablespoon Italian herb mix 1 cup tomato sauce

5 cups broth

1 cup corn

1   cup collard greens, torn into pieces

Directions:

1.   Put the olive oil until sizzling. Now, sauté the onion, sweet potatoes, bell pepper, carrots, parsnip, and celery until they've softened.

2.   Add in the garlic and continue sautéing for an additional 30 seconds.

3.   Now, add in the green lentils, Italian herb mix, tomato sauce, and vegetable broth; let it simmer for about 20 minutes until everything is thoroughly cooked.

4.   Add in the frozen corn and collard greens; cover and let it simmer for 5 minutes more.

Nutrition: Calories: 415, Fat: 6.6g, Carbs: 71g, Protein: 18.4g

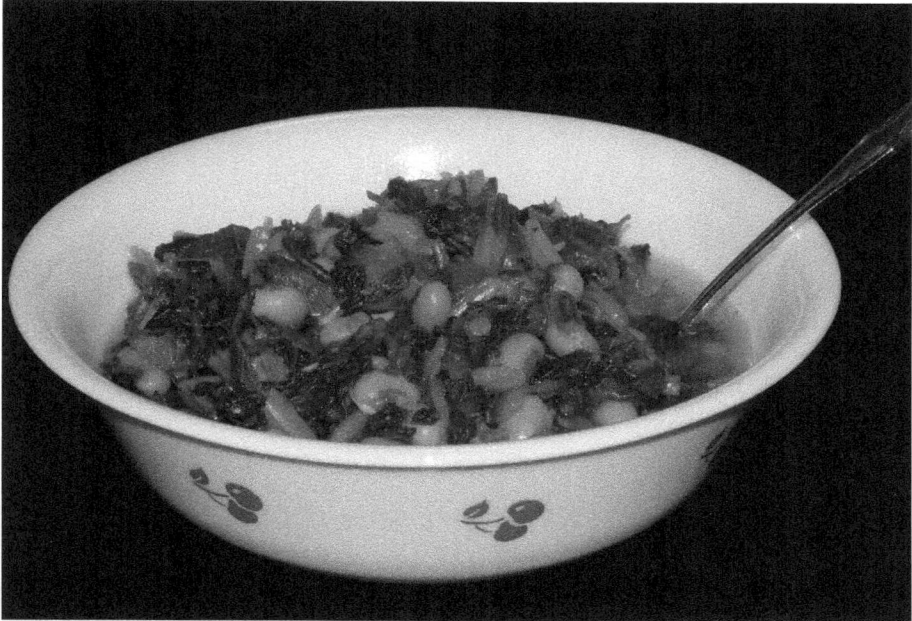

Chickpea Garden Vegetable Medley

Preparation Time: 10 minutes

Cooking Time: 10 minutes

Servings: 4

Ingredients:

2 tablespoons olive oil 1 onion, finely chopped 1 bell pepper, chopped 1 fennel bulb, chopped 3 cloves garlic, minced 2 ripe tomatoes, pureed

2 tablespoons fresh parsley, roughly chopped 2 tablespoons fresh basil, roughly chopped

2 tablespoons fresh coriander, roughly chopped 2 cups vegetable broth

14 oz. canned chickpeas, drained

Salt and pepper

1/2 teaspoon cayenne pepper

1 teaspoon paprika

1 avocado, peeled and sliced

Directions:

1.   Put the olive oil over medium heat. Once hot, sauté the onion, bell pepper, and fennel bulb for about 4 minutes.

2.   Sauté the garlic for about 1 minute or until aromatic.

3.   Add in the tomatoes, fresh herbs, broth, chickpeas, salt, black pepper, cayenne pepper, and paprika. Let it simmer, occasionally stirring, for about 20 minutes or until cooked through.

4.   Taste and adjust the seasonings. Serve garnished with the slices of the fresh avocado.

Nutrition: Calories: 369, Fat: 18.1g, Carbs: 43.5g, Protein: 13.2g

Hot Bean Dipping Sauce

Preparation Time: 10 minutes

Cooking Time: 10 minutes

Servings: 4

Ingredients:

2   (15-oz.) cans Great Northern beans, drained 2 tablespoons olive oil

2 tablespoons Sriracha sauce 2 tablespoons nutritional yeast 4 oz. vegan cream cheese

1/2 teaspoon paprika

1/2 teaspoon cayenne pepper 1/2 tsp

Salt and black pepper, to taste 4 oz. tortilla chips

Directions:

1.   Start by preheating your oven to 360°F.

2.   Pulse all the ingredients, except for the tortilla chips, in your food processor until your desired consistency is reached.

3.   Bake your dip in the preheated oven for about 25 minutes or until hot.

4.   Serve with tortilla chips and enjoy!

Nutrition: Calories: 175, Fat: 4.7g, Carbs: 24.9g, Protein: 8.8g

Chinese-Style Soybean Salad

Preparation Time: 10 minutes

Cooking Time: 10 minutes

Servings: 4

Ingredients:

1 (15-oz.) can soybeans, drained 1 cup arugula

1 cup baby spinach

1   cup green cabbage, shredded 1 onion, thinly sliced

1/2 tsp garlic

1 teaspoon ginger, minced

 1/2 teaspoon deli mustard 2 tablespoons soy sauce 1 tablespoon rice vinegar 1 tablespoon lime juice

2   tablespoons tahini

1 teaspoon agave syrup

Directions:

1.   In a salad bowl, place the soybeans, arugula, spinach, cabbage, and onion; toss to combine.

2.   In a small mixing dish, whisk the remaining ingredients for the dressing.

3.   Dress your salad and serve immediately.

Nutrition: Calories: 265, Fat: 13.7g, Carbs: 21g, Protein: 18g

Old-Fashioned Lentil and Vegetable Stew

Preparation Time: 10 minutes

Cooking Time: 10 minutes

Servings: 4

Ingredients:

3 tablespoons olive oil 1 large onion, chopped 1 carrot, chopped

1 bell pepper, diced

1 habanero pepper, chopped 3 cloves garlic, minced

Kosher salt and black pepper, to taste 1 teaspoon ground cumin

1 teaspoon smoked paprika

1 (28-oz.) can tomatoes, crushed 2 tablespoons tomato ketchup

4 cups vegetable broth

3/4 pound dry red lentils, soaked overnight and drained

1 avocado, sliced

Directions:

1.   Put the olive oil over medium heat. Once hot, sauté the onion, carrot, and peppers for about 4 minutes.

2.   Sauté the garlic for about 1 minute or so.

3.   Add in the spices, tomatoes, ketchup, broth, and canned lentils. Let it simmer, occasionally stirring, for about 20 minutes or until cooked through.

4.   Serve garnished with slices of avocado.

Nutrition: Calories: 475, Fat: 17.3g, Carbs: 61.4g, Protein: 23.7g

Indian Chana Masala

Preparation Time: 10 minutes

Cooking Time: 10 minutes

Servings: 4

Ingredients:

1 cup tomatoes, pureed

1 Kashmiri chile pepper, chopped 1 large shallot, chopped

1   tsp ginger, peeled and grated

4 tsp olive oil

2   cloves garlic, minced

1 teaspoon coriander seeds 1 teaspoon garam masala

1/2 teaspoon turmeric powder

Salt and pepper

1/2 cup vegetable broth

16 oz. canned chickpeas

1   tablespoon fresh lime juice

Directions

1.   In your blender or food processor, blend the tomatoes, Kashmiri chile pepper, shallot, and ginger into a paste.

2.   In a saucepan, heat the olive oil over medium heat. Once hot, cook the prepared paste and garlic for about 2 minutes.

3.   Add in the remaining spices, broth, and chickpeas. Turn the heat to a simmer. Continue to simmer for 8 minutes more or until cooked through.

4.   Remove from the heat. Drizzle fresh lime juice over the top of each serving.

Nutrition: Calories: 305, Fat: 17.1g, Carbs: 30.1g, Protein: 9.4g

Bok Choy Salad

Preparation Time: 10 minutes

Cooking Time: 10 minutes

Servings: 5

Ingredients:

10 oz bok choy, chopped

1 cup cherry tomatoes, halved

1 tablespoon black olives, pitted and sliced 1 mango, peeled and cubed

Juice of ½ orange

1 teaspoon curry powder 1 teaspoon sesame oil

1 tablespoon lemon juice

Directions:

1.   Add the bok choy, tomatoes, and the other ingredients to oil, toss and cook for 10 minutes.

2.   Divide into bowls and serve cold.

Nutrition: calories 142 fat 6.8 fiber 0.7 carbs 1.8 protein 9.4

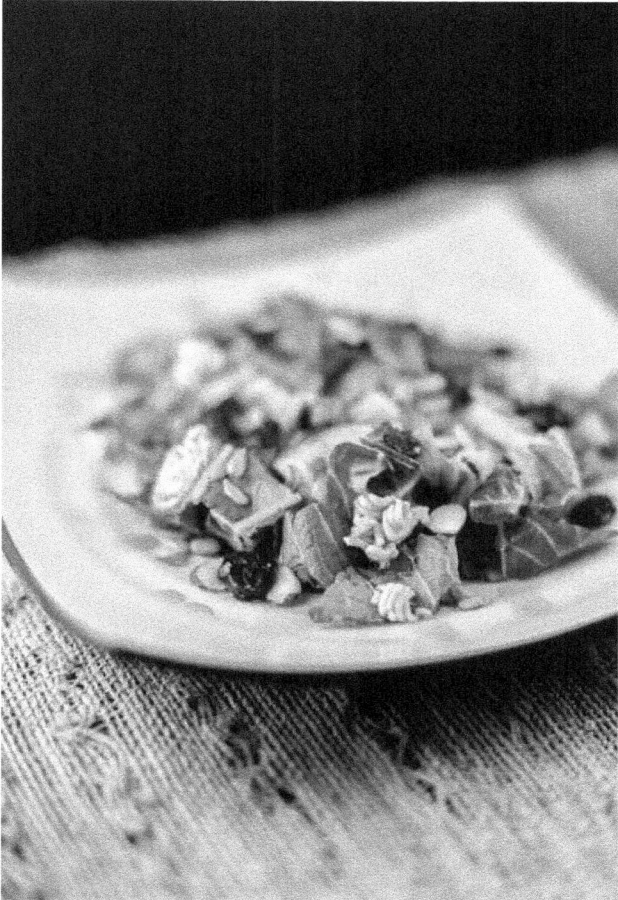

Balsamic Arugula and Beets

Preparation Time: 10 minutes

Cooking Time: 0 minutes

Servings: 4

Ingredients:

2 cups baby arugula

1   tablespoon balsamic vinegar 1 teaspoon olive oil

2   red beets, baked, peeled, and cubed 1 avocado, peeled, pitted, and cubed 1 teaspoon garam masala

½ teaspoon salt

½ teaspoon cayenne pepper

Directions:

1.   Mix arugula and beets and the other ingredients, toss and serve.

Nutrition: calories 151 fat 1.4 fiber 2.2 carbs 4.1 protein 5.9

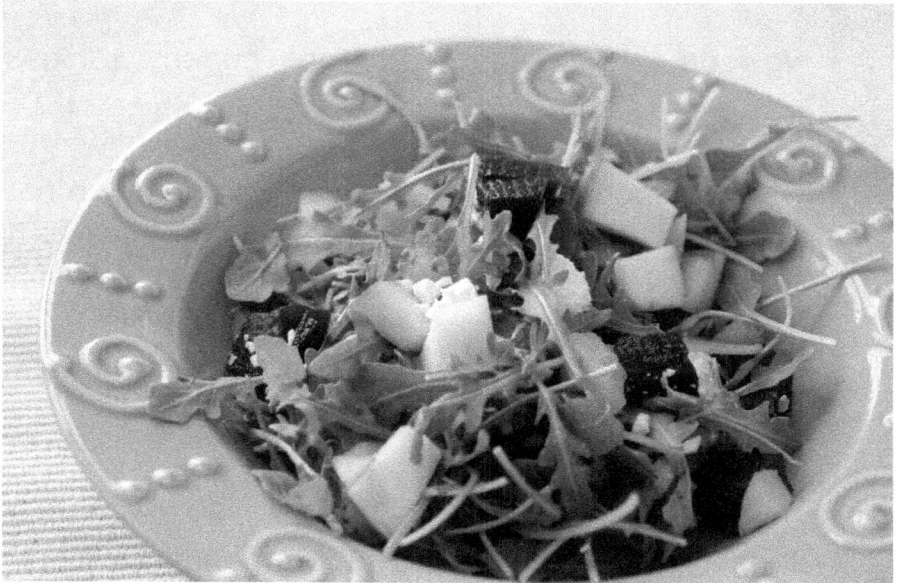

Herbed Beets

Preparation Time: 10 minutes

Cooking Time: 40 minutes

Servings: 3

Ingredients:

2 big red beets, peeled and roughly cubed 1 tablespoon chives, chopped

1   tablespoon cilantro, chopped 1 tablespoon basil, chopped Juice of 1 lime

A pinch of salt and black pepper

¼ teaspoon dried oregano

¼ teaspoon ground nutmeg

¼ teaspoon ground cumin 1 tablespoon olive oil

Directions:

1.   Spread the beets on a lined baking sheet, add the chives, cilantro, and the other ingredients, toss and bake at 400 degrees F for 40 minutes.

2.   Divide between plates and serve.

Nutrition: calories 188 fat 5.2 fiber 5.9 carbs 8.3 protein 1.6

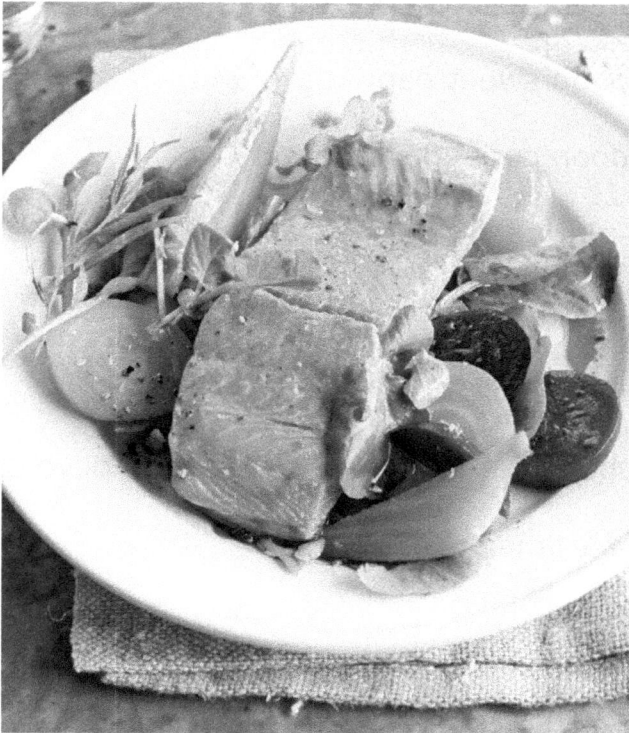

Marinara Broccoli

Preparation Time: 10 minutes

Cooking Time: 15 minutes

Servings: 4

Ingredients:

2   cups broccoli florets

1 teaspoon sweet paprika

1 teaspoon coriander, ground

¼ cup marinara sauce

½ teaspoon ground black pepper

½ teaspoon salt

½ teaspoon garlic powder 1 teaspoon olive oil

Juice of 1 lime

Directions: 1.   In a roasting pan, mix the broccoli with the marinara and the other ingredients, toss and bake at 400 degrees F for 15 minutes.

2. Divide between plates and serve.

Nutrition: calories206 fat 4.7 fiber 3.7 carbs 10.6 protein 6.1

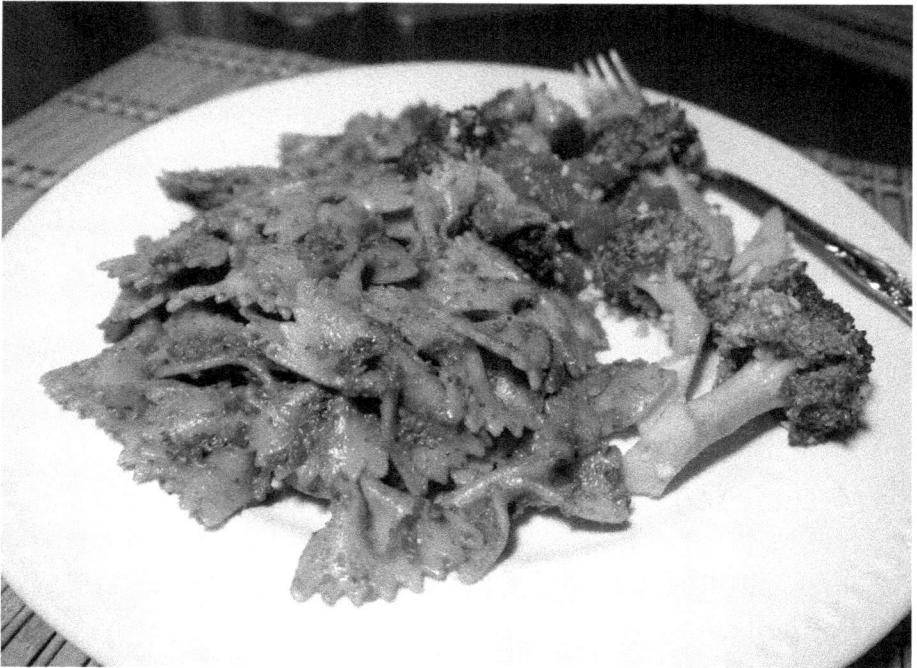

Spinach and Pear Salad

Preparation Time: 10 minutes

Cooking Time: 0 minutes

Servings: 2

Ingredients:

1   bell pepper, chopped

½ cup radishes halved

½ cup cherry tomatoes halved 2 cups baby spinach

2   and half pears, cored and cut into wedges 1 tablespoon walnuts, chopped

1 teaspoon chives, chopped

Salt and pepper

Juice of 1 lime

Directions:

1. In a bowl, mix the radishes with the pepper, tomatoes, and the other ingredients, toss and serve.

Nutrition: calories 143 fat 2.9 fiber 2.1 carbs 4.9 protein 3.2

Mango and Leeks Meatballs

Preparation Time: 20 minutes

Cooking Time: 10 minutes

Servings: 4

Ingredients:

1 tablespoon mango puree 1 cup leeks, chopped

½ cup tofu, crumbled

1 teaspoon dried oregano 1 tablespoon almond flour 1 teaspoon olive oil

1 tablespoon flax meal

½ teaspoon chili flakes

Directions:

1.   In the mixing bowl, mix up mango puree with leeks, tofu, and the other ingredients except for the oil and stir well.

2.   Make the small meatballs.

3.   After this, pour the olive oil into the skillet and heat it.

4.   Add the meatballs to the skillet and cook them for 4 minutes from each side.

Nutrition: calories 147 fat 8.6 fiber 4.5 carbs 5.6 protein 5.3

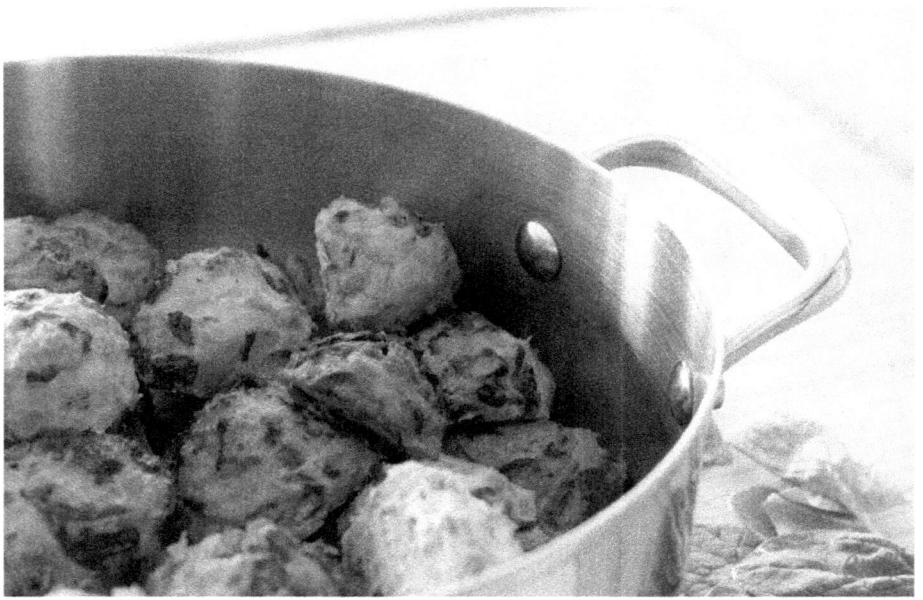

Spicy Carrots and Olives

Preparation Time: 15 minutes

Cooking Time: 10 minutes

Servings: 4

Ingredients:

½ teaspoon hot paprika

1 red chili pepper, minced

¼ teaspoon ground cumin

¼ teaspoon dried oregano

¼ teaspoon dried basil

½ teaspoon salt

1 tablespoon olive oil

1 pound baby carrots, peeled

1 cup olives

juice of 1 lime

Directions:

1.   Heat a pan with the oil over medium heat, add the carrots, olives, and the other ingredients, toss, cook for 10 minutes, divide between plates and serve.

Nutrition: calories 141 fat 5.8 fiber 4.3 carbs 7.5 protein 9.6

Harissa Mushrooms

Preparation Time: 15 minutes

Cooking Time: 30 minutes

Servings: 4

Ingredients:

1-pound mushroom caps 1 teaspoon harissa

1 teaspoon rosemary, dried 2 spring onions, chopped

1 leek, sliced

1   teaspoon thyme, dried 1 cup crushed tomatoes 1 teaspoon sweet paprika

A pinch of salt and black pepper 1 tablespoon olive oil

½ teaspoon lemon juice

Directions:

1.	In a roasting pan, mix the mushrooms with the harissa, rosemary, and the other ingredients and toss.

2.	Preheat the oven to 360F and put the pan inside.

3.	Cook the mix for 30 minutes, divide between plates and serve.

Nutrition: calories 250 fat 12.1 fiber 5.3 carbs 14.5 protein 12.9

Leeks and Artichokes Mix

Preparation Time: 10 minutes

Cooking Time: 30 minutes

Servings: 4

Ingredients:

2   cups artichoke hearts

3 leeks, sliced

1 cup cherry tomatoes, halved

¼ cup coconut cream

1 tablespoon almond flakes 1 teaspoon olive oil

1 teaspoon oregano, dried 1 teaspoon salt

1 teaspoon ground black pepper

¼ cup of chives, chopped

Directions:

1. Heat a pan with the oil over medium heat, add the leeks, oregano, salt, and pepper, stir and cook for 10 minutes.

2. Add artichokes and the other ingredients, toss, cook for 20 minutes, divide into bowls and serve.

Nutrition: calories 234 fat 9.7 fiber 4.2 carbs 9.6 protein 12.3

Coconut Avocado

Preparation Time: 10 minutes

Cooking Time: 0 minutes

Servings: 2

Ingredients:

2 avocados, halved, pitted, and roughly cubed 1 teaspoon dried thyme

2 tablespoons coconut cream

1   cup spring onions, chopped 1 teaspoon turmeric powder

Salt and black pepper to the taste

¼ teaspoon cayenne pepper

½ teaspoon onion powder

½ teaspoon garlic powder 1 teaspoon paprika

Salt and black pepper to the taste 2 tablespoons lemon juice

Directions:

1.   In a bowl, mix the avocados with the thyme, coconut cream, and the other ingredients, toss, divide between plates and serve.

Nutrition: calories 160 fat 6.9 fiber 7 carbs 12 protein 7

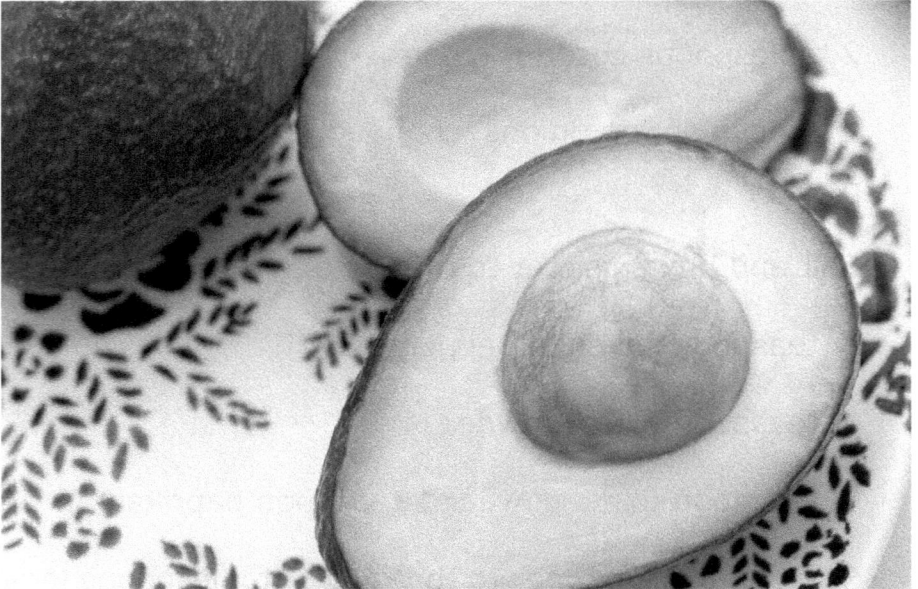

Red Kidney Bean Pâté

Preparation Time: 10 minutes

Cooking Time: 10 minutes

Servings: 4

Ingredients:

2   tablespoons oil

1 and half onion, chopped

1   bell pepper, chopped 2 cloves garlic, minced

2   cups red kidney beans, boiled and drained 1/4 cup olive oil

1   teaspoon stone-ground mustard

2   tablespoons fresh parsley, chopped 2 tablespoons fresh basil, chopped

Salt and pepper, to taste

Directions:

1.   In a saucepan, heat the olive oil over medium-high heat. Now, cook the onion, pepper, and garlic until just tender or about 3 minutes.

2.   Add the sautéed mixture to your blender; add in the remaining ingredients. Puree the ingredients in your blender or food processor until smooth and creamy.

Nutrition:

Calories: 135, Fat: 12.1g, Carbs: 4.4g, Protein: 1.6g

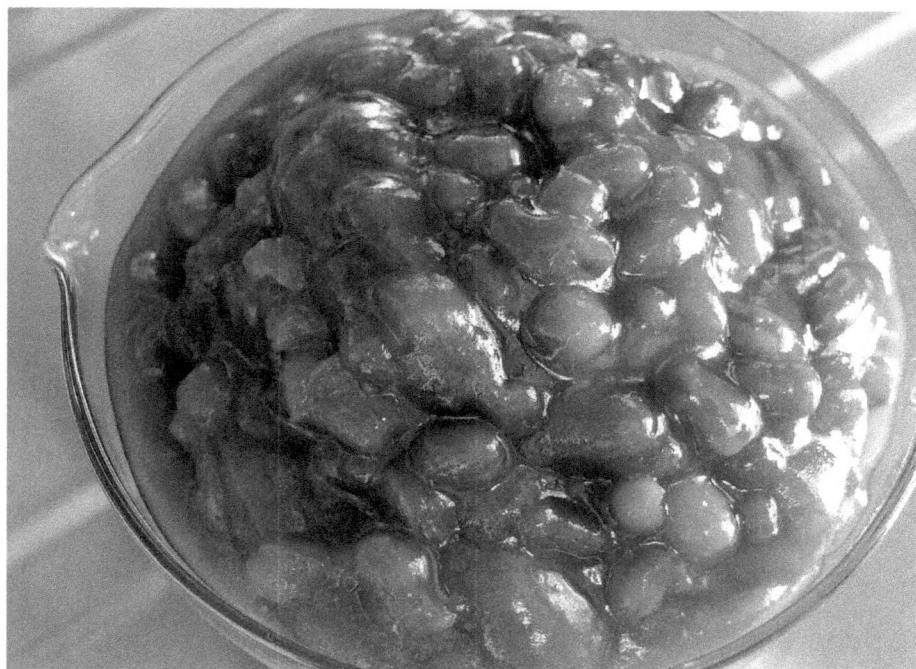

Brown Lentil Bowl

Preparation Time: 10 minutes

Cooking Time: 10 minutes

Servings: 4

Ingredients:

1   cup brown lentils, soaked overnight, and drained
3 cups water

2   cups brown rice, cooked 1 zucchini, diced

1 red onion, chopped

1 teaspoon garlic, minced 1 cucumber, sliced

1 bell pepper, sliced

4 tablespoons olive oil

1   tablespoon rice vinegar 2 tablespoons lemon juice
2 tablespoons soy sauce

1/2 teaspoon dried oregano 1/2 teaspoon cumin

Salt and pepper

2 cups arugula

2   cups Romaine lettuce, torn into pieces

Directions:

1.   Add the brown lentils and water to a saucepan and bring to a boil over high heat. Then, turn the heat to a simmer and continue to cook for 20 minutes or until tender.

2.   Let lentils cool completely.

3.   Add in the remaining ingredients and toss to combine well. Serve at room temperature or well-chilled

Nutrition: Calories: 452, Fat: 16.6g, Carbs: 61.7g, Protein: 16.4g

Hot and Spicy Anasazi Bean Soup

Preparation Time: 10 minutes

Cooking Time: 10 minutes

Servings: 4

Ingredients:

2 cups Anasazi beans, soaked overnight, drained, and rinsed 8 cups water

2   bay leaves

3   tablespoons olive oil

2 medium onions, chopped 2 bell peppers, chopped

1 habanero pepper, chopped

3 cloves garlic, pressed or minced

Sea salt and pepper, to taste

Directions

1.   In a soup pot, bring the Anasazi beans and water to a boil. Once boiling, turn the heat to a simmer. Add

in the bay leaves and let it cook for about 1 hour or until tender.

2.   Meanwhile, in a heavy-bottomed pot, heat the olive oil over medium-high heat. Now, sauté the onion, peppers, and garlic for about 4 minutes until tender.

3.   Add the sautéed mixture to the cooked beans. Season with salt and black pepper.

4.   Continue to simmer, stirring periodically, for 10 minutes more or until everything is cooked through.

Nutrition: Calories: 352, Fat: 8.5g, Carbs: 50.1g, Protein: 19.7g

Black-Eyed Pea Salad (Ñebbe)

Preparation Time: 10 minutes

Cooking Time: 10 minutes

Servings: 4

Ingredients:

2 cups peas, soaked and drained

2 tbsp basil leaves, chopped

2 tablespoons parsley leaves, chopped 1 shallot, chopped

1   cucumber, sliced

2   bell peppers, seeded and diced

1 Scotch bonnet chili pepper, seeded and finely chopped

 1 cup cherry tomatoes, quartered

Salt and pepper, to taste

2 tablespoons fresh lime juice

1 tbsp apple cider vinegar

1/4 cup extra-virgin olive oil

1 avocado, peeled, pitted, and sliced

Directions:

1.   Cover the black-eyed peas with water by 2 inches and bring to a gentle boil. Let it boil for about 15 minutes.

2.   Then, turn the heat to a simmer for about 45 minutes. Let it cool completely.

3.   Place the black-eyed peas in a salad bowl. Add in the basil, parsley, shallot, cucumber, bell peppers, cherry tomatoes, salt, and black pepper.

4.   In a mixing bowl, whisk the lime juice, vinegar, and olive oil.

5.   Dress the salad, garnish with fresh avocado and serve immediately.

Nutrition: Calories: 471, Fat: 17.5g, Carbs: 61.5g, Protein: 20.6g

Middle Eastern Za'atar Hummus

Preparation Time: 10 minutes

Cooking Time: 10 minutes

Servings: 4

Ingredients:

10 oz. chickpeas, boiled and drained 1/4 cup tahini

2 tablespoons extra-virgin olive oil

2 tablespoons sun-dried tomatoes, chopped 1 lemon, freshly squeezed

2 garlic cloves, minced

Salt and pepper, to taste

1/2 teaspoon smoked paprika

1   teaspoon Za'atar

Directions:

1.   Mix all the ingredients until creamy and uniform.

2.   Place in your refrigerator until ready to serve.

Nutrition: Calories: 140, Fat: 8.5g, Carbs: 12.4g, Protein: 4.6g

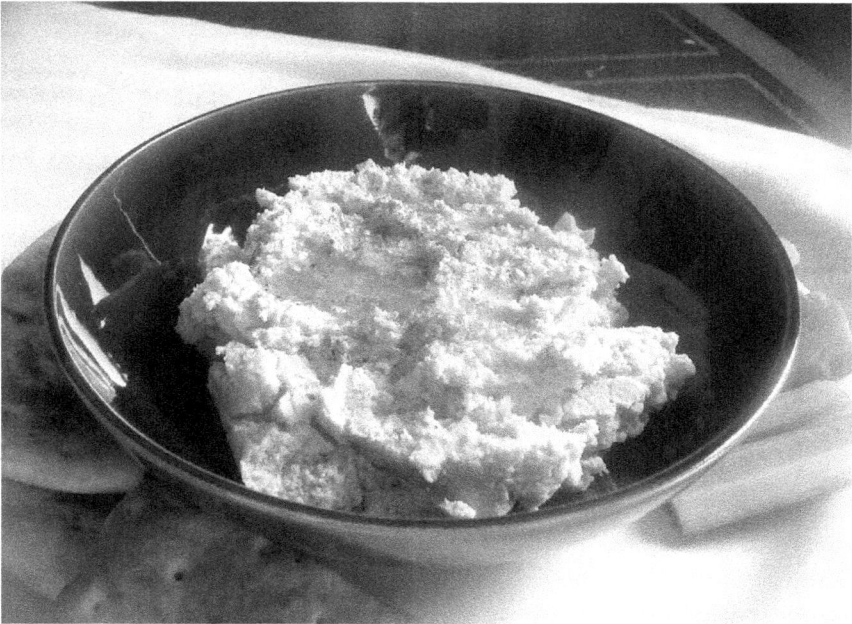

Black Bean Pizza

Preparation Time: 30 minutes

Cooking Time: 20 minutes

Servings: 2

Ingredients:

1 Sliced avocado 1 Sliced red onion 1 Grated carrot

1 Sliced tomato

5 cup Spicy black bean dip 2 Pizza crusts

Directions:

1.   Turn on the oven and let heat to 400 degrees. Layout two crusts on a baking sheet and add the dip onto each one.

2.   Top with the tomato slices and sprinkle the carrots and the onion on a well.

3.   Add to the oven and let it bake for about 20 minutes or so until done. Top with the avocado before serving.

Nutrition: Calories: 379 Carbs: 59g Fat: 13g Protein: 13g

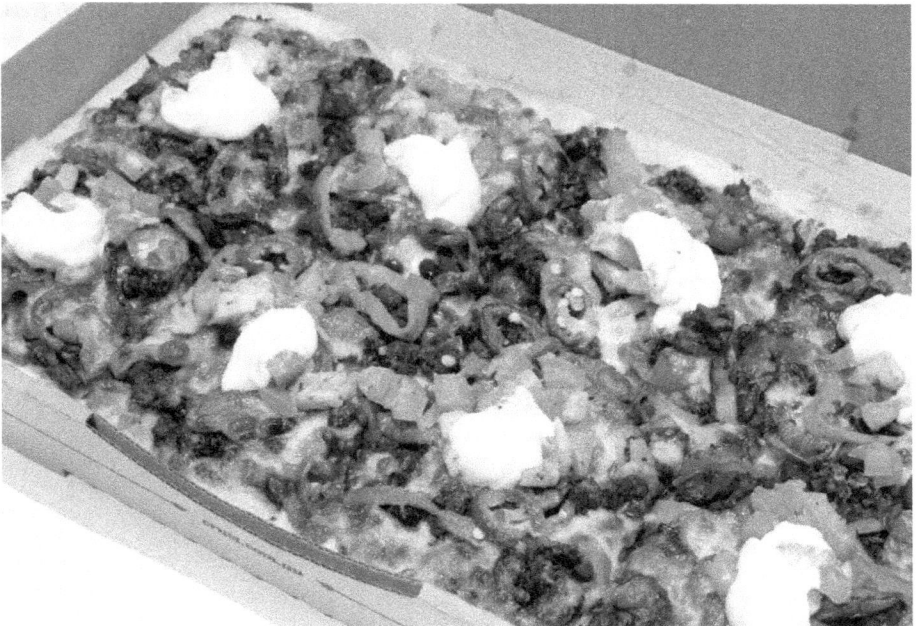

Vegetable and Chickpea Loaf

Preparation Time: 10 minutes

Cooking Time: 15 minutes

Servings: 4

Ingredients:

1 tsp. Salt

5 tsp. Dried sage 1 tsp. Dried savory 1 tbsp. Soy sauce

25 cup Parsley

5 cup Breadcrumbs

75 cup oats

75 cup Chickpea flour

1.5 cup cooked chickpeas 2 Minced garlic cloves

1 Chopped yellow onion 1 Shredded carrot

1 Shredded white potato

Directions:

1.   Set the oven to 350F. Take out a loaf pan and then grease it up.

2.   Squeeze out the liquid from the potato and add to the food processor with garlic, onion, and carrot.

3.   Add the chickpeas and pulse to blend well. Add in the rest of the ingredients here, and when it is done, use your hands to form this into a loaf and add to the pan.

4.   Place into the oven to bake for a bit until it is nice and firm. Let it cool down, and then slice.

Nutrition: Calories: 351 kcal Protein: 16.86 g Fat: 6.51 g Carbohydrates: 64 g

Thyme and Lemon Couscous

Preparation Time: 5 minutes

Cooking Time: 10 minutes

Servings: 6

Ingredients:

25 cup Chopped parsley

1.5 cup Couscous

2   tbsp. Chopped thyme Juice and zest of a lemon

2.75 cup Vegetable stock

Directions:

1.   Take out a pot and add in the thyme, lemon juice, and vegetable stock. Stir in the couscous after it has gotten to a boil, and then take off the heat.

2.   Allow sitting covered until it can take in all of the liquid. Then fluff up with a form.

Nutrition: Calories: 922 kcal Protein: 2.7 g Fat: 101.04 g Carbohydrates: 10.02 g

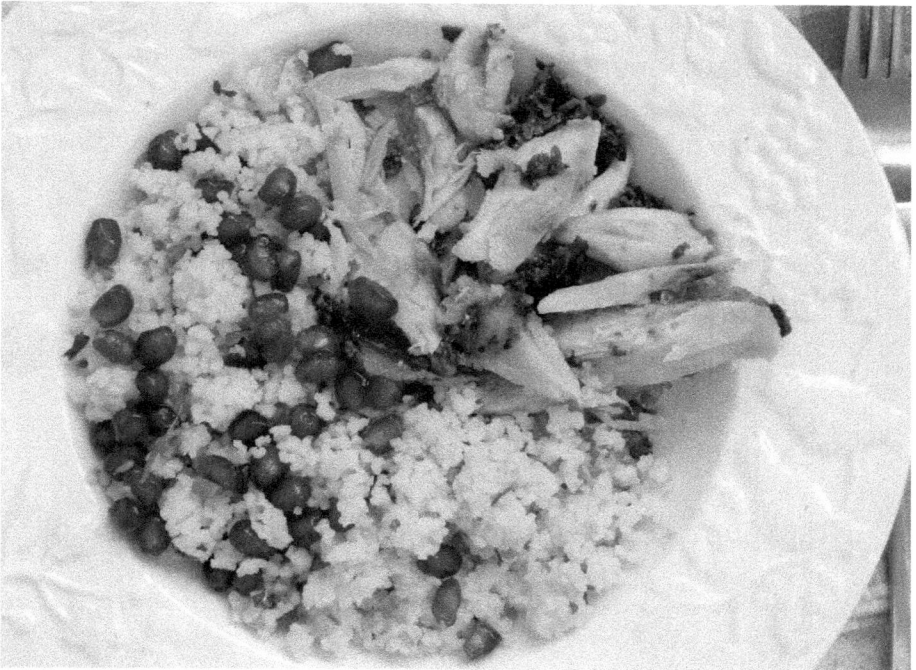

Olives and Mango Mix

Preparation Time: 10 minutes

Cooking Time: 0 minutes

Servings: 2

Ingredients:

1 cup black olives, pitted and halved

1 cup olive

1 cup mango, peeled and cubed

Salt and pepper

Juice of 1 lime

1 teaspoon sweet paprika

1 teaspoon coriander, ground 1 tablespoon olive oil

Directions:

1.   In a bowl, mix the olives with the mango and the other ingredients, toss and serve.

Nutrition: calories 68 fat 4.4 fiber 0 carbs 1.5 protein 3.3

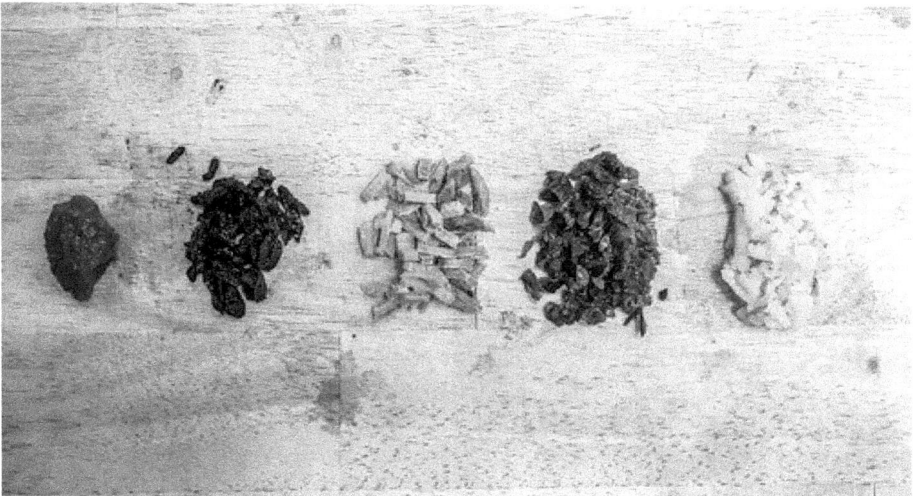

Eggplant and Avocado Mix

Preparation Time: 10 minutes

Cooking Time: 20 minutes

Servings: 4

Ingredients:

1   pound eggplant, roughly cubed

2   avocados, peeled, pitted, and cubed

1 red onion, chopped

1 tsp curry powder

Juice of 1 lime

½ cup crushed tomatoes 1 tablespoon olive oil

1 teaspoon salt

1   teaspoon chili powder

Directions:

1.   Add onion to oil and cook for 5 minutes.

2.   Add the eggplants, avocados, and the other ingredients, toss and cook for 15 minutes more.

3.   Divide between plates and serve.

Nutrition: calories 231 fat 7.6 fiber 8.5 carbs 9.2 protein 5.4

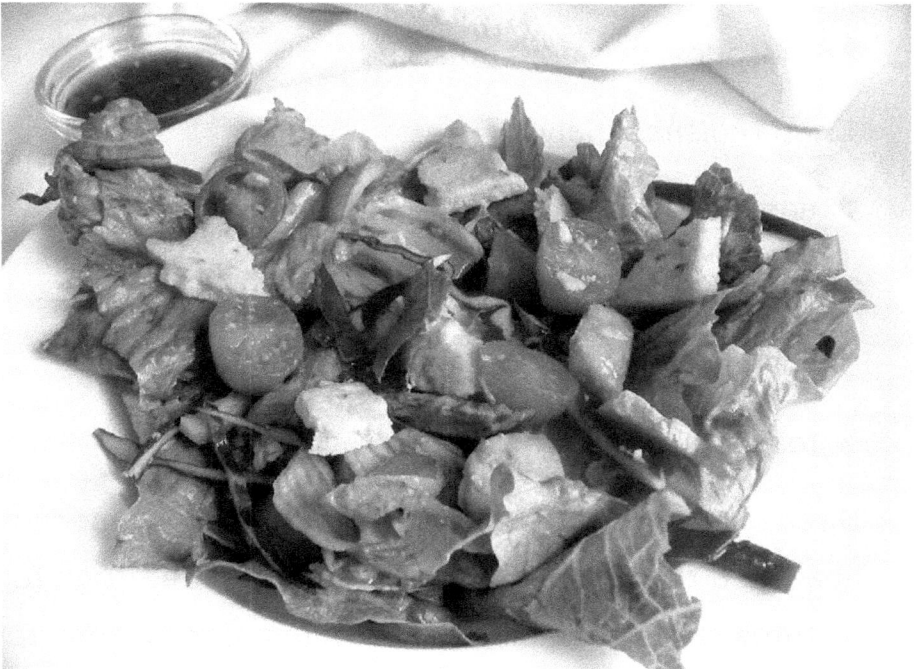

Red Onion, Avocado, and Radishes Mix

Preparation Time: 15 minutes

Cooking Time: 12 minutes

Servings: 2

Ingredients:

2   red onions, peeled

2 avocados, peeled, and sliced

1 cup radishes, halved

1 teaspoon oregano, dried 1 teaspoon basil, dried

1 tbsp olive oil

1 tsplemon juice

¼ teaspoon salt

Directions: 1.   Heat a pan with the oil over medium heat, add the onions, oregano, and basil and cook for 5 minutes. 2. Add remainings ingredients, toss, cook for 7 minutes more, divide into bowls and serve.Nutrition: calories 145 fat 7.1 fiber 2.4 carbs 10.3 protein 6.2

Cajun and Balsamic Okra

Preparation Time: 10 minutes

Cooking Time: 15 minutes

Servings: 2

Ingredients:

1 cup okra, sliced

½ cup crushed tomatoes

1   teaspoon Cajun seasoning

2   tablespoons balsamic vinegar 1 teaspoon salt

1 teaspoon ground black pepper

1 tablespoon fresh parsley, chopped 1 teaspoon olive oil

Directions:

1.   Heat a pan with the oil over medium heat, add the okra, seasoning, and the remaining ingredients, toss and cook for 15 minutes.

2.   Divide into bowls and serve.

Nutrition: calories 162 fat 4.5 fiber 4.6 carbs 12.6
protein 3

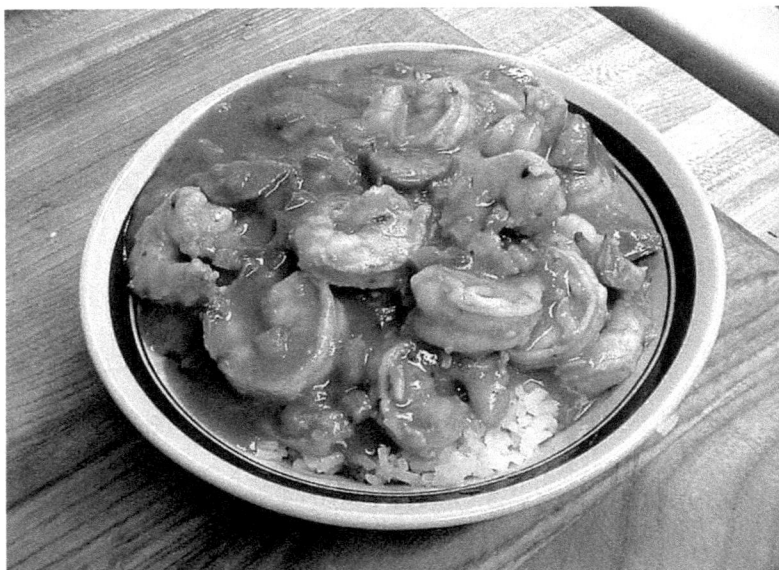

Mexican Chickpea Taco Bowls

Preparation Time: 10 minutes

Cooking Time: 10 minutes

Servings: 4

Ingredients:

2 tablespoons sesame oil 1 red onion, chopped

1   habanero pepper, minced 2 garlic cloves, crushed

2   bell peppers, seeded and diced Sea salt and ground black pepper 1/2 teaspoon Mexican oregano

1 teaspoon ground cumin 2 ripe tomatoes, pureed

1 teaspoon brown sugar

16 oz. canned chickpeas drained 4 (8-inch) flour tortillas

2   tablespoons fresh coriander, roughly chopped

Directions:

1.   In a large skillet, heat the sesame oil over moderately high heat. Then, sauté the onions for 2 to 3 minutes or until tender.

2.   Add in the peppers and garlic and continue to sauté for 1 minute or until fragrant.

3.   Add in the spices, tomatoes, and brown sugar and bring to a boil. Immediately turn the heat to a simmer, add in the canned chickpeas and let it cook for 8 minutes longer or until heated through.

4.   Toast your tortillas and arrange them with the prepared chickpea mixture.

5.   Top with fresh coriander and serve immediately.

Nutrition: Calories: 409, Fat: 13.5g, Carbs: 61.3g, Protein: 13.8g

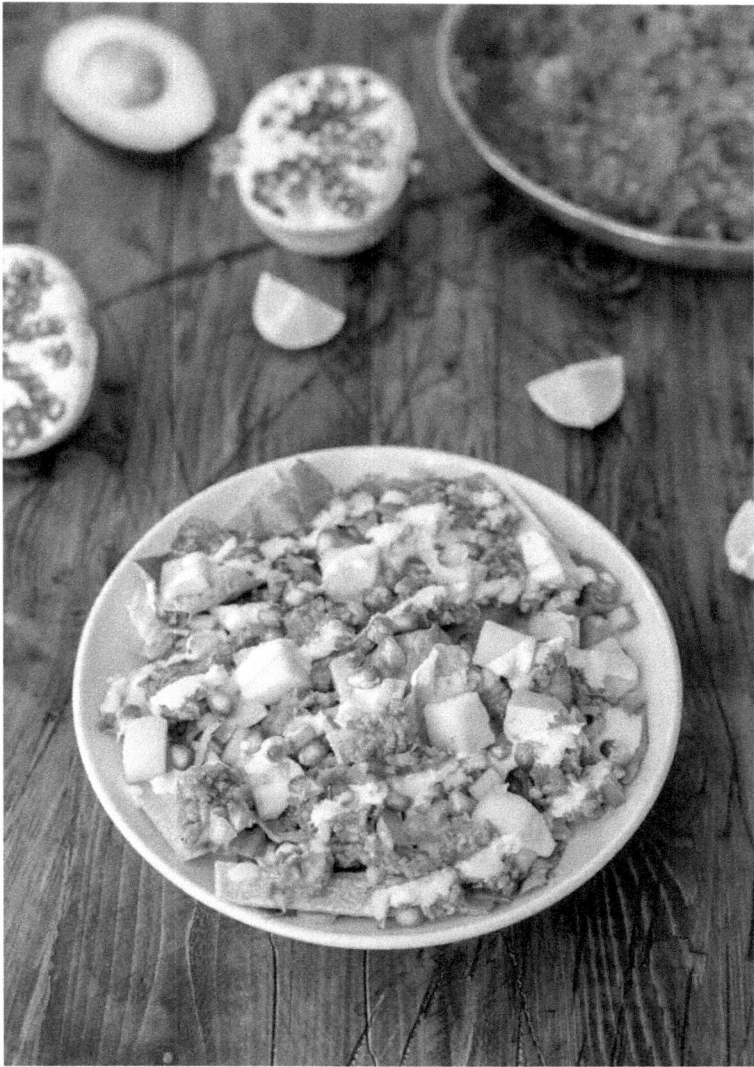

Indian Dal Makhani

Preparation Time: 10 minutes

Cooking Time: 10 minutes

Servings: 4

Ingredients:

3   tablespoons sesame oil 1 large onion

1 pepper

2 garlic cloves, minced

1   tablespoon ginger, grated

2   chilies

1 tsp cumin seeds

1 bay laurel

1 teaspoon turmeric powder 1/4 teaspoon red peppers 1/4 teaspoon ground allspice 1/2 teaspoon garam masala 1 cup tomato sauce

4 cups vegetable broth

1 ½ cups black lentils, soaked overnight and drained 4-5 curry leaves for garnish

Directions:

1. Sauté the onion and bell pepper for 3 minutes more until they've softened.

2.   Add in the garlic, ginger, green chilies, cumin seeds, and bay laurel; continue to sauté, frequently stirring, for 1 minute or until fragrant.

3.   Add the ingredients. Now, turn the heat to a simmer. Cook for 12 minutes more.

4.   Garnish with curry leaves and serve hot!

Nutrition: Calories: 329, Fat: 8.5g, Carbs: 44.1g, Protein: 16.8g

Mexican-Style Bean Bowl

Preparation Time: 10 minutes

Cooking Time: 10 minutes

Servings: 4

Ingredients:

1   pound red beans, soaked overnight and drained 1 cup canned corn kernels, drained

2   roasted bell peppers, sliced 1 chili pepper, finely chopped 1 cup cherry tomatoes, halved 1 red onion, chopped

1/4 cup cilantro

1/4 cup fresh parsley, chopped 1 teaspoon Mexican oregano 1/4 cup red wine vinegar

2 tablespoons fresh lemon juice 1/3 cup extra-virgin olive oil

Sea salt and ground black, to taste 1 avocado, peeled, pitted, and sliced

Dire ns:

over the soaked beans with a fresh change of
1
iter and bring to a boil. Let it boil for about 10
s. Turn the heat to a simmer and continue to
or 50 to 55 minutes or until tender.

Allow your beans to cool completely, then transfer
to a salad bowl.

. Add in the remaining ingredients and toss to
combine well. Serve at room temperature.

Nutrition: Calories: 465, Fat: 17.9g, Carbs: 60.4g,
Protein: 20.2g

Classic Italian Minestrone

Preparation Time: 10 minutes

Cooking Time: 10 minutes

Servings: 4

Ingredients:

2 tbsp olive oil

1 onion, diced

2 carrots, sliced

4   cloves garlic, minced 1 cup elbow pasta

5   cups vegetable broth

1 (15-oz.) can white beans, drained 1 large zucchini, diced

1 (28-oz.) can tomatoes, crushed

1 tablespoon fresh oregano leaves, chopped 1 tablespoon fresh basil leaves, chopped

1   tablespoon fresh Italian parsley, chopped

Directions:

1.   Put the olive oil until sizzling. Now, sauté the onion and carrots until they've softened.

2.   Add in the garlic, uncooked pasta, and broth; let it simmer for about 15 minutes.

3.   Stir in the beans, zucchini, tomatoes, and herbs. Continue to cook, covered, for about 10 minutes until everything is thoroughly cooked.

4.   Garnish with some extra herbs, if desired.

Nutrition: Calories: 305, Fat: 8.6g, Carbs: 45.1g, Protein: 14.2g

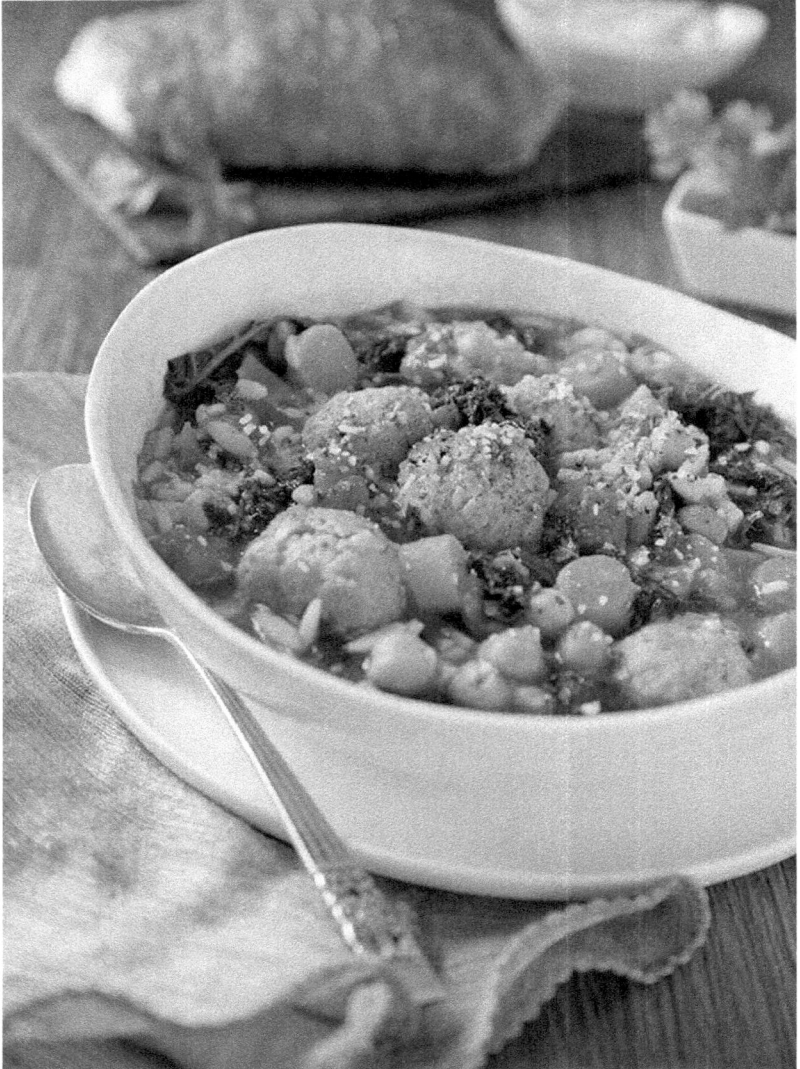

www.ingramcontent.com/pod-product-compliance
Lightning Source LLC
Chambersburg PA
CBHW070722030426
42336CB00013B/1889